Your Pancreatic Journey

I0427444

Surprising Insights and Revealed Truths
to Pancreatic Health

Dr. Richard Nuel

Copyright

Table Of Content

Acknowledgements

As the author of this journey through the landscape of pancreatic diseases, my heart is brimming with gratitude for those who've illuminated the path. Foremost, I extend my deepest thanks to the healthcare warriors and patients who shared their stories of resilience and hope, teaching me the true essence of strength. To the medical experts who generously lent their knowledge, ensuring accuracy and compassion in every page, your guidance was indispensable. My family and friends, your unwavering support was my anchor in turbulent times. This book, a beacon for those navigating the stormy seas of illness, is a testament to your collective spirit and generosity.

Introduction

The Journey Ahead: Understanding and Living with Pancreatic Diseases

Embarking on a journey with pancreatic disease can feel like navigating through uncharted waters, where the horizon is clouded with uncertainty and fear. This book, "The Journey Ahead: Understanding and Living with Pancreatic Diseases," is your compass and map, designed to guide you through the complexities of these conditions, illuminating paths of knowledge, support, and hope.

Pancreatic diseases, encompassing a range of disorders from acute and chronic pancreatitis to pancreatic cancer, affect thousands of individuals worldwide, yet they remain shrouded in mystery and misconceptions. The intent of this book is to dispel the fog of uncertainty, offering clear, accessible information that demystifies these conditions. By understanding the workings of the pancreas, the signs and symptoms of its ailments, and the latest in treatment options, patients and their loved ones can navigate their diagnosis with confidence and grace.

But this journey is not solely about medical facts and figures. It's about the human spirit, the challenges of living with a chronic condition, and the resilience required to face each day. It's about finding community, seeking support, and sharing in the collective wisdom of those who've walked this path before you. Through personal stories, expert advice, and practical tips for daily living, this book aims to be a source of comfort and strength, encouraging you to take an active role in your care and advocating for a life filled with quality and joy, despite the hurdles.

As you turn these pages, remember that you are not alone on this journey. There is a vast community of patients, caregivers, and medical professionals walking alongside you, each step of the way.

How to Use This Book

This book is designed as a comprehensive guide for patients, caregivers, and anyone touched by the spectrum of pancreatic diseases. It serves multiple purposes: to educate, to comfort, and to empower. Whether you're seeking a deep understanding of pancreatic conditions, looking for management strategies, or in need of emotional support, you'll find sections tailored to your journey. Start by reading the introductory chapters to grasp the basics of pancreatic functions and the impact of diseases on this vital organ. From there, navigate to the chapters that correspond to your specific condition for detailed insights into symptoms, diagnosis, treatment options, and managing daily life.

Each chapter is structured to provide both medical information and personal stories, offering a balance of professional guidance and real-world experiences. The management sections outline practical advice for dietary adjustments, lifestyle changes, and coping mechanisms, while the emotional support sections offer strategies for mental health and building a support network.

Use the appendices for quick reference to nutritional advice, a glossary of medical terms, and a directory of resources and support services. Remember, this book is not just to be read but to be used actively as a companion in your journey towards understanding, managing, and living with pancreatic disease.

Chapter 1

The Pancreas Unveiled

The Role of the Pancreas in Your Body

The pancreas, a vital but often overlooked organ nestled deep within the abdomen, plays a pivotal role in the body's digestive and endocrine systems. This slender, pear-shaped organ, bridging the gap between the stomach and the spine, is a powerhouse of metabolic activity, crucial for maintaining our health and well-being. "The Pancreas Unveiled" chapter aims to shed light on this enigmatic organ, elucidating its functions and the critical role it plays in our body.

Primarily, the pancreas serves two main functions: an exocrine role, aiding in digestion, and an endocrine role, regulating blood sugar levels. The exocrine part of the pancreas produces digestive enzymes, which are secreted into the small intestine to break down fats, proteins, and carbohydrates, facilitating the absorption of nutrients. Without these enzymes, our body would be unable to extract the vital nourishment needed from the food we consume.

Simultaneously, the pancreas performs an equally crucial endocrine function. It houses the Islets of Langerhans, clusters of cells that produce hormones like insulin and glucagon. Insulin plays a fundamental role in lowering blood sugar levels by facilitating the uptake of glucose by cells for energy production. Glucagon, on the other hand, works in opposition to insulin, raising blood sugar levels by prompting the liver to release stored glucose. This delicate balance maintained by the pancreas ensures our body's energy homeostasis, keeping our blood sugar levels within a narrow, healthy range.

Understanding the pancreas's dual role illuminates why diseases affecting this organ can have profound impacts on both digestion and glucose metabolism, leading to complex health challenges. By unveiling the functions and importance of the pancreas, we begin to appreciate the intricate ballet of hormones and enzymes it orchestrates, a testament to the complexity and resilience of the human body. This foundational knowledge is crucial for anyone looking to understand the impact of pancreatic diseases and underscores the importance of this often-underestimated organ in our overall health.

When Things Go Wrong: An Overview of Pancreatic Diseases

When the pancreas, a critical organ for digestion and blood sugar regulation, malfunctions, it can lead to a spectrum of pancreatic diseases, each with its own set of challenges and implications for health. Pancreatic diseases can broadly be classified into acute conditions, like acute pancreatitis, which is often a sudden and severe inflammation that can be life-threatening if not treated promptly; and chronic conditions, such as chronic pancreatitis and pancreatic cancer, which have long-lasting effects and can significantly impact quality of life.

Acute pancreatitis typically arises from gallstones blocking the ducts of the pancreas or excessive alcohol consumption, leading to severe abdominal pain, nausea, and vomiting. Chronic pancreatitis, on the other hand, results from prolonged inflammation, leading to permanent damage and a decrease in the organ's ability to function properly, causing digestive problems and diabetes.

Pancreatic cancer, one of the most aggressive forms of cancer, is particularly insidious because it often remains undetected until it's in an advanced stage, making treatment difficult. Symptoms like jaundice, weight loss, and abdominal pain usually appear late in the disease process.

Furthermore, conditions such as pancreatic insufficiency and cystic fibrosis affect the pancreas's ability to produce enzymes or hormones necessary for digestion and glucose regulation, leading to malnutrition and diabetes. Understanding these diseases is crucial for early detection, effective management, and improving patient outcomes.

Chapter 2

Navigating the Diagnosis

Recognizing the Symptoms: When to Seek Help

Navigating the path to a diagnosis for pancreatic diseases can be fraught with uncertainty, given the organ's deep abdominal location and the often subtle or complex nature of its symptoms. Recognizing the symptoms early and understanding when to seek medical help are critical steps in securing a timely diagnosis and initiating effective treatment.

Symptoms of pancreatic diseases can vary widely depending on the specific condition but often include persistent abdominal pain that may radiate to the back, unexplained weight loss, jaundice (yellowing of the skin

15

and eyes), changes in stool, nausea, and vomiting. Acute symptoms, such as severe abdominal pain accompanied by fever or a rapid pulse, demand immediate medical attention.

Chronic symptoms, like ongoing digestive issues or new-onset diabetes without clear risk factors, also warrant evaluation. Importantly, early stages of pancreatic cancer and other pancreatic diseases may not cause symptoms, making regular check-ups and discussing any changes in health with a healthcare provider crucial.

Knowing your body and being vigilant about changes is essential. If symptoms persist or impact your quality of life, it's imperative to consult a healthcare professional. Early detection is key in managing pancreatic diseases effectively, and recognizing when to seek help can make a significant difference in outcomes.

The Diagnostic Process: Tests and What They

Mean

The diagnostic process for pancreatic diseases involves a series of steps and tests, each playing a crucial role in determining the nature and extent of the condition.

Understanding these tests and their implications is vital for patients navigating their diagnostic journey.

Initial evaluation typically begins with a thorough medical history and physical examination, where healthcare providers look for signs such as jaundice, abdominal tenderness, or unexpected weight loss. Blood tests are often the next step, measuring enzyme levels like amylase and lipase, which can indicate pancreatitis, or checking for tumor markers in cases of suspected pancreatic cancer.

Imaging tests provide a more detailed view of the pancreas and surrounding structures. Ultrasound may be used as a first-line imaging tool, but more detailed images can be obtained with a CT scan or MRI, which can identify inflammation, tumors, or blockages in the pancreas. Endoscopic ultrasound (EUS) combines endoscopy and ultrasound to get closer views of the pancreas, and can also be used to take biopsy samples.

In some cases, an ERCP (Endoscopic Retrograde Cholangiopancreatography) may be performed to examine the pancreatic and bile ducts, especially if blockages or stones are suspected.

Each test contributes a piece to the puzzle, helping healthcare providers formulate a diagnosis and tailor a treatment plan that addresses the specific needs of the patient. Understanding these tests and their purposes empowers patients to actively participate in their care.

Interpreting Medical Jargon: A Glossary for the

Newly Diagnosed

For those newly diagnosed with a pancreatic disease, the medical terminology can seem like an overwhelming barrage of jargon. To bridge this gap, an essential tool is a glossary that demystifies medical terms, making the diagnostic and treatment process more comprehensible. Here's a concise overview:

- Pancreas: A gland behind the stomach, involved in both digestion and blood sugar regulation.
- Acute Pancreatitis: Sudden inflammation of the pancreas, often marked by severe abdominal pain.
- Chronic Pancreatitis: Long-term inflammation that leads to permanent damage and decreased function.
- Pancreatic Cancer: A malignant tumor of the pancreas, often diagnosed at a late stage due to subtle early symptoms.
- Jaundice: Yellowing of the skin and eyes, typically caused by liver problems or blockages affecting bile flow.

- Amylase and Lipase: Enzymes measured in blood tests to assess pancreatic function; elevated levels may indicate pancreatitis.
- CT Scan/MRI: Imaging tests providing detailed pictures of the pancreas and surrounding tissues, useful in identifying tumors or inflammation.
- Endoscopic Ultrasound (EUS): A procedure combining endoscopy and ultrasound to examine the digestive tract and pancreas.
- ERCP (Endoscopic Retrograde Cholangiopancreatography): A technique used to study the pancreatic and bile ducts, and sometimes to remove blockages.

This glossary is a starting point to help newly diagnosed patients navigate discussions with healthcare providers, fostering a better understanding of their condition and care pathway.

Chapter 3

Acute Pancreatitis

Understanding Acute Pancreatitis

Acute pancreatitis is a sudden inflammation of the pancreas, an organ critical to digestion and glucose regulation. This condition arises when digestive enzymes become active inside the pancreas, attacking and damaging its tissues. This can cause severe abdominal pain, nausea, vomiting, and, in more severe cases, lead to systemic complications affecting the heart, lungs, and kidneys.

The primary triggers for acute pancreatitis include gallstones and excessive alcohol consumption. Gallstones can block the pancreatic duct, leading to enzyme buildup and inflammation. Similarly, alcohol can directly damage pancreatic cells and also lead to duct obstruction. Other causes might include medications, high triglyceride levels, and abdominal trauma.

Symptoms typically manifest as a sudden, severe pain in the upper abdomen that may radiate to the back, often accompanied by fever, a swollen and tender abdomen, nausea, and vomiting. Diagnosis is usually confirmed through a combination of blood tests showing elevated levels of pancreatic enzymes, and imaging tests like CT scans or MRIs that visualize inflammation or blockages.

Treatment focuses on resting the pancreas, managing pain, preventing dehydration, and addressing the underlying cause. In mild cases, acute pancreatitis can resolve with a few days of hospital care, but severe instances may require more intensive treatment. Recognizing and promptly addressing symptoms of acute pancreatitis can significantly affect outcomes, emphasizing the importance of early intervention.

Medical Treatments and Interventions

Medical treatments and interventions for pancreatic diseases aim to alleviate symptoms, manage complications, and improve the patient's quality of life. The choice of treatment depends on the specific pancreatic condition, its severity, and individual patient factors. Here are some common medical treatments and interventions:

1. Pain Management: Pain is a significant symptom of pancreatic diseases. Medications, such as nonsteroidal anti-inflammatory drugs (NSAIDs) and opioids, may be prescribed to manage pain. In some cases, nerve blocks or celiac plexus neurolysis can provide relief.

2. Enzyme Replacement Therapy (ERT): Patients with pancreatic insufficiency may require ERT to aid in the digestion of food. Pancreatic enzyme supplements are taken with meals to help break down fats, proteins, and carbohydrates.

3. Nutritional Support: Nutritional deficiencies are common in pancreatic diseases. Nutritional support may include dietary modifications, enteral nutrition through a feeding tube, or total parenteral nutrition (TPN) for severe cases.

4. Endoscopic Procedures: Endoscopy can be used to treat conditions such as pancreatic pseudocysts or blockages. Endoscopic retrograde cholangiopancreatography (ERCP) can help clear obstructions in the pancreatic or bile ducts.

5. Surgery: Surgical interventions may be necessary for conditions like pancreatic cancer, chronic pancreatitis, or pseudocysts. Procedures can range from tumor removal (pancreatectomy) to drainage of pseudocysts.

6. Chemotherapy and Radiation: For pancreatic cancer, chemotherapy and radiation therapy may be recommended either before or after surgery to shrink tumors or target cancer cells.

7. Immunotherapy: Emerging treatments like immunotherapy are being explored in clinical trials for pancreatic cancer. These therapies harness the immune system to fight cancer cells.

8. Diabetes Management: If diabetes develops as a result of pancreatic disease, medications, insulin therapy, or lifestyle modifications may be prescribed to manage blood sugar levels.

9. Palliative Care: In advanced cases, palliative care focuses on improving the patient's comfort and quality of life, addressing symptoms, and providing emotional support.

10. Clinical Trials: Participation in clinical trials can offer access to cutting-edge treatments and therapies for pancreatic diseases, contributing to ongoing research.

Treatment plans are individualized, and a multidisciplinary healthcare team, including gastroenterologists, surgeons, oncologists, dietitians, and pain specialists, collaborates to provide the best possible care. Patients and caregivers should actively engage with their healthcare providers to make informed decisions about treatment options.

Managing Your Recovery at Home

Managing your recovery at home is a crucial aspect of living with pancreatic diseases. It empowers patients to take an active role in their healthcare and enhances their overall well-being. Here are key strategies for managing your recovery at home:

1. Medication Adherence: Follow your prescribed medication regimen diligently. Set reminders if necessary and communicate any side effects or concerns with your healthcare provider.

2. Dietary Modifications: If you have dietary restrictions, adhere to your recommended diet plan. This may include low-fat, easily digestible meals, enzyme replacement therapy, and adequate hydration.

3. Monitor Symptoms: Keep a symptom diary to track changes in pain, appetite, bowel movements, and overall health. Share this information with your healthcare team during appointments.

4. Hydration: Staying well-hydrated is essential. Sip water throughout the day, especially if you experience diarrhea or vomiting.

5. Pain Management: Follow your pain management plan as prescribed by your healthcare provider. Report any changes in pain levels promptly.

6. Nutritional Supplements: If advised, take nutritional supplements or vitamins to address deficiencies and support your overall health.

7. Activity and Rest: Strike a balance between rest and light physical activity. Gentle exercises like walking can help maintain strength and energy levels.

8. Emotional Well-being: Seek emotional support through support groups, therapy, or speaking with a counselor if you're struggling with the emotional aspects of your condition.

9. Follow-up Appointments: Attend all follow-up appointments with your healthcare team. These visits

are essential for monitoring your progress and adjusting your treatment plan as needed.

10. Emergency Plan: Have an emergency plan in place, including contact information for healthcare providers and instructions on what to do in case of severe symptoms or complications.

11. Family and Caregiver Support: Engage your family and caregivers in your recovery plan. Their support can make a significant difference in your journey.

12. Education: Continuously educate yourself about your condition and treatment options. Informed patients can actively participate in their care decisions.

Managing your recovery at home is a collaborative effort between you, your healthcare team, and your support network. By adhering to your treatment plan, maintaining a healthy lifestyle, and seeking the necessary support, you can optimize your recovery and enhance your quality of life while living with pancreatic diseases.

Real Stories: The Road to Recovery

Real stories from individuals who have navigated the road to recovery from pancreatic diseases provide not only a source of inspiration but also invaluable insights into the personal challenges and triumphs faced along the way. One such story is of Alex, who was diagnosed with acute pancreatitis after experiencing severe abdominal pain. Initially overwhelmed by the diagnosis, Alex found strength through the support of healthcare professionals and a community of patients with similar experiences. Through a combination of hospitalization for immediate care, followed by lifestyle adjustments and strict dietary changes, Alex gradually regained strength and control over his health.

Another inspiring story comes from Jordan, who battled chronic pancreatitis for years. Jordan's journey was marked by persistent pain and multiple hospital visits, but the turning point came with a tailored treatment plan that included enzyme replacement therapy and pain management strategies. Jordan also engaged in a patient support group, finding solace and understanding among peers.

These stories underscore the importance of a comprehensive approach to recovery, involving medical

27

intervention, lifestyle modifications, and emotional support. They highlight the resilience of the human spirit and the power of community, offering hope to those embarking on their own journeys of recovery from pancreatic diseases.

Chapter 4

Chronic Pancreatitis

Living with Chronic Pancreatitis

Living with chronic pancreatitis presents a complex challenge, demanding adjustments to daily life and ongoing management to mitigate symptoms and maintain quality of life. Chronic pancreatitis is a long-term inflammation of the pancreas that leads to irreversible damage over time, affecting the organ's ability to function properly. Patients often experience persistent abdominal pain, malabsorption of nutrients, and the development of diabetes as the pancreas loses its ability to produce insulin.

The condition requires a multifaceted approach to management, including dietary changes, enzyme supplementation to aid digestion, and pain management strategies. Nutrition plays a critical role; a low-fat diet, small frequent meals, and avoidance of alcohol can help manage symptoms and prevent flare-ups. Enzyme replacement therapy is often necessary to improve nutrient absorption and minimize gastrointestinal symptoms.

Pain management is another crucial aspect, with options ranging from medication to more invasive procedures for those with severe pain. Additionally, patients may need to manage diabetes with insulin therapy as part of their treatment plan.

Living with chronic pancreatitis also involves addressing the emotional and psychological impacts of the disease. Support groups, mental health counseling, and patient education are essential components of care, helping individuals navigate the challenges of chronic illness and maintain a hopeful outlook on life.

Nutritional Management and Lifestyle Changes

Nutritional management and lifestyle changes play pivotal roles in managing pancreatic diseases, offering patients a proactive way to influence their health outcomes positively. For those dealing with conditions like chronic pancreatitis or pancreatic insufficiency, adapting dietary habits can significantly alleviate symptoms, improve nutrient absorption, and enhance overall well-being.

A key element of nutritional management involves tailoring the diet to reduce the pancreas's workload and prevent malnutrition. This typically includes eating low-fat meals, as fat can be particularly challenging for the compromised pancreas to digest. Small, frequent meals are recommended over large, heavy ones to ease the digestive process. Incorporating easily digestible foods rich in proteins and carbohydrates, while limiting difficult-to-digest fats, helps maintain energy levels and supports healing.

Lifestyle changes extend beyond diet alone. Reducing or eliminating alcohol consumption is crucial, as alcohol can exacerbate pancreatic conditions. Smoking cessation is also recommended, as smoking increases the risk of pancreatitis and pancreatic cancer. Regular, gentle exercise can support digestion and help manage symptoms like fatigue and stress.

Moreover, staying hydrated is essential, especially for those experiencing frequent vomiting or diarrhea, to prevent dehydration. These nutritional and lifestyle adjustments, coupled with medical treatment, form a comprehensive approach to managing pancreatic diseases, emphasizing the power of diet and lifestyle in the journey toward health and stability.

Pain Management Strategies

Pain management is a critical component of the treatment plan for individuals suffering from pancreatic diseases, particularly those with chronic pancreatitis, where pain can be a persistent and debilitating symptom. Effective pain management strategies are multifaceted, aiming not only to alleviate pain but also to improve the patient's overall quality of life.

Medications are often the first line of defense in pain management, with options ranging from non-opioid analgesics for mild pain to more potent opioids for severe discomfort. However, due to the risks of long-term opioid use, including dependency and tolerance, their use is carefully monitored and typically reserved for cases where other treatments have failed.

For some patients, endoscopic or surgical interventions may provide relief by addressing the underlying causes of pain, such as obstructed pancreatic ducts. Techniques like endoscopic pancreatic duct stenting or decompression, and surgical procedures like the

Puestow procedure, can significantly reduce pain by improving pancreatic drainage.

In addition to medical interventions, lifestyle modifications play a crucial role in pain management. Dietary changes, such as adopting a low-fat diet and small, frequent meals, can minimize pancreatic stimulation and reduce pain. Complementary therapies, including acupuncture, yoga, and physical therapy, can also be beneficial in managing chronic pain, offering patients a holistic approach to their condition. Integrating these strategies requires a personalized approach, often involving a multidisciplinary team to address the physical, emotional, and psychological aspects of living with pancreatic disease.

Emotional Coping Mechanisms

Emotional coping mechanisms are essential for individuals navigating the challenges of pancreatic diseases, as the psychological impact of chronic illness can be as daunting as the physical symptoms. Recognizing and addressing the emotional toll is crucial for maintaining mental health and overall well-being.

One effective coping mechanism is seeking support, whether through formal counseling or support groups.

Sharing experiences with others who understand the journey can provide comfort, reduce feelings of isolation, and offer practical advice for managing the condition. Professional therapists specializing in chronic illness can also help individuals develop strategies to cope with anxiety, depression, and the stress of living with a long-term health condition.

Mindfulness and stress-reduction techniques, such as meditation, deep breathing exercises, and yoga, can also be beneficial. These practices help individuals stay present, reduce anxiety, and manage pain through relaxation techniques. Engaging in hobbies and activities that bring joy and fulfillment can also serve as a distraction from pain and illness, contributing to a positive outlook on life.

Additionally, maintaining open communication with family, friends, and healthcare providers about one's feelings and struggles fosters a support network that can provide encouragement and assistance when needed. Adopting these emotional coping mechanisms enables individuals to navigate the complexities of their condition with resilience and strength, enhancing their capacity to manage both the physical and emotional aspects of pancreatic diseases.

Chapter 5

Pancreatic Cancer

Facing Pancreatic Cancer: An Overview

Pancreatic cancer, one of the most formidable challenges in the realm of gastrointestinal malignancies, presents a daunting journey for those diagnosed. This type of cancer arises when cells in the pancreas, an organ pivotal to digestion and blood sugar regulation, begin to grow uncontrollably. Due to its tendency to remain asymptomatic in the early stages, pancreatic cancer often goes undetected until it has advanced, complicating treatment efforts and affecting prognosis.

Risk factors for pancreatic cancer include smoking, chronic pancreatitis, diabetes, obesity, and a family history of the disease. Symptoms, when they do appear, may include jaundice, abdominal pain, weight loss, and loss of appetite, prompting the need for a thorough evaluation.

Diagnosis typically involves a combination of imaging tests, such as CT scans or MRIs, and may include biopsy procedures to confirm the presence of cancer cells. Treatment options are determined based on the stage of the cancer and can include surgery, chemotherapy, radiation therapy, or a combination of these approaches. Surgery, when feasible, offers the best chance for a cure but is often only an option in early-stage disease.

Despite the challenges, advances in treatment and supportive care offer hope, improving the quality of life and survival rates for many patients facing pancreatic cancer. It's a journey of resilience, requiring comprehensive care and support from a multidisciplinary medical team, alongside the unwavering support of loved ones.

Treatment Pathways: Surgery, Chemotherapy, and Radiation

Treatment pathways for pancreatic diseases, particularly pancreatic cancer, encompass a multidisciplinary approach tailored to the individual's condition, stage of disease, and overall health. Surgery, chemotherapy, and radiation therapy are the primary modalities used, either alone or in combination, to manage the disease and improve patient outcomes.

Surgery is often the first-line treatment for pancreatic cancer, provided the cancer is localized and resectable. Procedures such as the Whipple operation remove the affected part of the pancreas, along with a portion of the stomach, small intestine, and other nearby tissues. This approach aims to remove the cancer entirely but is only an option for a minority of patients at diagnosis due to the typically advanced stage of the disease at presentation.

Chemotherapy involves the use of drugs to kill cancer cells or stop them from growing and dividing. It can be administered before surgery (neoadjuvant chemotherapy) to shrink tumors, making them easier to remove, or after surgery (adjuvant chemotherapy) to

37

eliminate any remaining cancer cells, thereby reducing the risk of recurrence.

Radiation therapy uses high-energy rays to target and destroy cancer cells. It can be used as a standalone treatment, in combination with chemotherapy (chemoradiation), or as a palliative treatment to relieve symptoms in advanced cases.

The choice among these treatments depends on a comprehensive evaluation of the disease's specifics and the patient's condition, aiming to achieve the best possible quality of life and survival outcomes.

Navigating Life During Treatment

Navigating life during treatment for pancreatic diseases, especially cancer, involves adjusting to a new normal that encompasses medical appointments, treatment sessions, and managing side effects. It's a period marked by physical, emotional, and often financial challenges, requiring resilience and a robust support system to maintain quality of life.

Patients may experience a range of side effects from treatments such as chemotherapy and radiation, including fatigue, nausea, changes in appetite, and susceptibility to infections. These effects necessitate modifications in daily routines, with an emphasis on rest, nutrition, and self-care. Adopting a balanced diet, staying hydrated, and engaging in light exercise as tolerated can help manage treatment side effects and maintain strength.

Emotional and psychological support is equally vital. Many find solace in counseling, support groups, or therapy, which provide a safe space to share experiences and coping strategies. Open communication with healthcare providers about the challenges faced during treatment is crucial for receiving the necessary support and adjustments to treatment plans.

Financial considerations are also a significant aspect of navigating life during treatment, with many facing the burden of medical bills and possibly reduced income. Exploring resources for financial assistance, such as through cancer support organizations, can alleviate some of this stress.

Throughout this journey, it's important to focus on small victories and moments of joy, leaning on loved ones and healthcare professionals for support and guidance.

Support for the Soul: Emotional and Psychological Care

Support for the soul through emotional and psychological care is a critical aspect of managing life with pancreatic diseases, particularly for those facing the daunting challenge of pancreatic cancer. The diagnosis and treatment journey can evoke a whirlwind of emotions, including fear, anger, sadness, and isolation. Addressing these feelings is just as important as managing the physical symptoms of the disease.

Emotional and psychological care involves a comprehensive approach that includes counseling, support groups, and sometimes medication to manage depression or anxiety. Professional counselors or psychologists specializing in chronic illness can provide valuable strategies for coping with the emotional rollercoaster of diagnosis, treatment, and the uncertainties of living with a serious health condition.

Support groups play a crucial role in emotional care, offering a sense of community and understanding. Sharing experiences with others who are facing similar challenges can significantly reduce feelings of isolation and despair, fostering a supportive environment where patients and caregivers can find comfort and hope.

Mindfulness practices, such as meditation and yoga, can also be beneficial, helping individuals to remain present and find peace amidst the turmoil of their disease. These practices promote relaxation, reduce stress, and improve mental health, contributing to a holistic approach to emotional and psychological well-being.

Chapter 6

Pancreatic Insufficiency

Understanding Pancreatic Insufficiency: Causes and Effects

Pancreatic insufficiency is a condition characterized by the pancreas's inability to produce enough enzymes necessary for the proper digestion and absorption of nutrients from food. This insufficiency can lead to malabsorption, resulting in nutritional deficiencies and weight loss, as the body fails to obtain essential vitamins, fats, proteins, and carbohydrates from the diet.

The primary cause of pancreatic insufficiency is chronic pancreatitis, a condition marked by persistent inflammation that leads to the destruction of pancreatic tissue over time. Other causes may include cystic fibrosis, pancreatic surgery, or hereditary disorders affecting the pancreas. These conditions disrupt the pancreas's normal function, reducing its enzyme-producing capabilities and affecting its contribution to the digestive process.

The effects of pancreatic insufficiency are multifaceted, impacting not only nutritional status but also overall health and quality of life. Symptoms may include steatorrhea (fatty stools), weight loss, abdominal discomfort, and diarrhea. Because the body cannot absorb nutrients efficiently, patients may experience fatigue, weakness, and an increased risk of osteoporosis and vitamin deficiencies.

Managing pancreatic insufficiency typically involves enzyme replacement therapy (ERT), where patients take pancreatic enzyme supplements with meals to aid digestion. Dietary adjustments and nutritional support are also crucial to address malabsorption issues and ensure adequate intake of nutrients.

Treatment Options and Digestive Enzyme Replacement Therapy

Treatment options for pancreatic insufficiency primarily focus on addressing the enzyme deficiency that impedes proper digestion and absorption of nutrients. The cornerstone of managing this condition is Digestive Enzyme Replacement Therapy (ERT), which involves taking pancreatic enzyme supplements with meals and snacks to mimic the enzymes the pancreas would normally produce. These supplements contain a mix of lipase, protease, and amylase, which are essential for breaking down fats, proteins, and carbohydrates, respectively.

The goal of ERT is to improve nutritional absorption, thereby alleviating symptoms of malabsorption such as steatorrhea (fatty, loose stools), weight loss, and vitamin deficiencies. The effectiveness of enzyme replacement therapy is closely monitored through patient symptoms and nutritional status, with dosage adjustments made based on the fat content of meals and the individual's specific needs.

In addition to ERT, patients with pancreatic insufficiency may benefit from dietary modifications, such as consuming smaller, more frequent meals and limiting dietary fat intake to reduce the digestive burden on the pancreas. Vitamins and mineral supplements, particularly fat-soluble vitamins (A, D, E, and K), may also be prescribed to address specific nutritional deficiencies.

Collaboration with a healthcare team, including gastroenterologists and nutritionists, is essential for optimizing the management of pancreatic insufficiency, ensuring that treatment strategies are tailored to each patient's unique situation and needs.

Dietary Adjustments and Lifestyle Management

Dietary adjustments and lifestyle management play a crucial role in the overall treatment plan for individuals with pancreatic diseases, especially those suffering from conditions like chronic pancreatitis or pancreatic insufficiency. A well-considered diet can significantly alleviate symptoms, improve nutrient absorption, and enhance quality of life.

For those affected, dietary adjustments often involve adopting a low-fat diet to ease the pancreas's workload and reduce symptoms such as abdominal pain and steatorrhea. Patients are advised to consume small, frequent meals throughout the day instead of large, heavy meals, which can overburden the digestive system. Incorporating easily digestible foods rich in proteins and carbohydrates, while minimizing difficult-to-digest fats, helps ensure adequate nutrition.

In addition to dietary changes, lifestyle management includes abstaining from alcohol and smoking, as these can exacerbate pancreatic conditions. Regular, moderate exercise is encouraged to support overall health and aid digestion. Staying hydrated is also vital, particularly for individuals experiencing frequent vomiting or diarrhea.

Collaboration with healthcare professionals, including dietitians who specialize in gastrointestinal disorders, is essential for creating a personalized diet plan. This collaborative approach ensures that dietary adjustments and lifestyle changes are practical, sustainable, and tailored to meet the individual's specific needs and preferences, thereby optimizing the management of pancreatic diseases.

Patient Stories: Adapting to Life with Pancreatic Insufficiency

Patient stories about adapting to life with pancreatic insufficiency highlight the resilience and adaptability required to manage this challenging condition. One such story is of Maria, who was diagnosed with pancreatic insufficiency following a long battle with chronic pancreatitis. Initially overwhelmed by the dietary restrictions and the necessity of taking enzyme supplements with every meal, Maria found solace in the support of online communities and patient groups. Through sharing experiences and tips, she learned to navigate her new dietary landscape, finding creative ways to enjoy her meals while adhering to her nutritional needs.

Then there's John, who after his diagnosis, struggled with the symptoms of malabsorption, leading to significant weight loss and fatigue. The turning point came when he began working with a dietitian specializing in pancreatic disorders. Together, they devised a meal plan that catered to his caloric and nutritional requirements, incorporating enzyme therapy effectively. John's story is a testament to the importance of personalized care and the positive impact of dietary management on quality of life.

These narratives underscore the individual journeys of those living with pancreatic insufficiency, reflecting the initial challenges of diagnosis, the learning curve associated with dietary and lifestyle adjustments, and ultimately, the triumph of adapting to a new normal. They serve as a beacon of hope and a source of practical advice for others embarking on a similar journey.

Chapter 7

Pancreatic Pseudocysts

The Basics of Pancreatic Pseudocysts

Pancreatic pseudocysts are fluid-filled sacs that form in the abdomen as a complication of pancreatic inflammation, typically resulting from acute pancreatitis or chronic pancreatitis. Unlike true cysts, which are lined by epithelium, pseudocysts are surrounded by fibrous tissue and lack a true epithelial lining, hence the prefix "pseudo." These cysts arise due to the accumulation of pancreatic enzymes, blood, and necrotic tissue following pancreatic duct disruption or pancreatic tissue damage.

Pseudocysts can vary in size and may present with symptoms or remain asymptomatic, depending on their size and location. When symptoms do occur, they can include abdominal pain, bloating, nausea, vomiting, and, in some cases, jaundice if the cyst compresses the bile duct. The diagnosis of pancreatic pseudocysts typically involves imaging studies such as CT scans, MRI, or endoscopic ultrasound (EUS), which help to visualize the cyst's structure and determine its relation to surrounding pancreatic tissue and ducts.

Management of pancreatic pseudocysts depends on the symptoms, size, and presence of complications. Asymptomatic pseudocysts may be monitored for changes, while symptomatic pseudocysts often require intervention. Treatment options include endoscopic drainage, where the fluid is drained through the stomach or duodenum wall using endoscopic techniques, or, less commonly, surgical removal for larger or complicated pseudocysts.

Interventional Treatments: Drainage Procedures

and Surgical Options

Interventional treatments for conditions such as pancreatic pseudocysts and abscesses are vital, focusing on drainage procedures and, when necessary, surgical options to relieve symptoms and prevent complications.

Drainage of pancreatic pseudocysts can be achieved through various techniques, each chosen based on the cyst's characteristics and patient's overall health.

Endoscopic drainage is a preferred method for many, utilizing endoscopic ultrasound (EUS) to guide the insertion of a stent into the cyst, allowing it to drain into the stomach or duodenum. This minimally invasive approach offers the advantages of reduced recovery time and lower risk of complications compared to traditional surgery.

For pseudocysts that are not amenable to endoscopic drainage or in cases where endoscopic approaches have failed, percutaneous catheter drainage may be considered. Under imaging guidance, a catheter is placed through the skin into the pseudocyst to facilitate drainage externally.

In more complex cases, or when pseudocysts are associated with necrosis or infection, surgical options may be necessary. Surgical drainage, such as cystogastrostomy or cystojejunostomy, involves creating a connection between the pseudocyst and the stomach or jejunum to allow for continuous drainage. These procedures are more invasive and typically reserved for situations where less invasive methods are not feasible or have been unsuccessful.

Each interventional treatment is tailored to the individual's specific condition, with the goal of alleviating symptoms, promoting healing, and minimizing the risk of complications.

Monitoring and Managing Pseudocysts at Home

Monitoring and managing pancreatic pseudocysts at home requires vigilance and adherence to care plans prescribed by healthcare providers. While interventional treatments may be necessary for some pseudocysts, many can be managed conservatively, especially if they are asymptomatic or if they present with mild symptoms.

Patients with pancreatic pseudocysts should be educated on recognizing signs that indicate changes in their condition. Symptoms such as increasing abdominal pain, fever, jaundice, changes in bowel habits, or signs of infection should prompt immediate medical consultation. Regular follow-up appointments are crucial for tracking the pseudocyst's size and assessing any potential complications through imaging tests like ultrasound or CT scans.

Dietary management plays a significant role in home care, with patients often advised to adopt a low-fat diet to reduce the pancreas's workload and avoid exacerbating symptoms. Staying well-hydrated and eating small, frequent meals can also help manage discomfort and support overall digestive health.

Patients should also be counseled on the importance of avoiding alcohol and smoking, as these can aggravate pancreatic conditions and hinder the healing process. Engaging in gentle physical activity, as tolerated, can promote overall well-being and aid in recovery.

Personal Experiences: Overcoming Challenges with Pseudocysts

Personal experiences with pancreatic pseudocysts often highlight the resilience required to overcome the challenges posed by this condition. One such story comes from Emma, who was diagnosed with a large pseudocyst following an episode of acute pancreatitis. Initially overwhelmed by the diagnosis, Emma faced significant abdominal pain and digestive issues. Through a combination of careful monitoring, dietary adjustments, and close communication with her healthcare team, she managed to navigate the complexities of her condition. Emma's journey included an endoscopic drainage procedure, which significantly alleviated her symptoms and allowed her to gradually return to her daily activities.

Another story is of Liam, who experienced recurrent pseudocysts that impacted his quality of life. Determined to find a long-term solution, Liam underwent a more invasive surgical intervention to remove the pseudocyst. Post-surgery, he focused on his recovery, adhering to a strict diet and gradually increasing his physical activity. Liam's experience underscores the importance of persistence and the willingness to explore different treatment options in consultation with medical professionals.

These personal stories illuminate the varied paths to managing and overcoming the challenges of pancreatic pseudocysts. They highlight the importance of patient education, proactive management, and the support of a multidisciplinary healthcare team in achieving positive outcomes.

Chapter 8

Rare Pancreatic Disorders

Pancreatic Neuroendocrine Tumors (PNETs): A

Different Kind of Enemy

Pancreatic Neuroendocrine Tumors (PNETs) represent a distinct category within the spectrum of pancreatic disorders, differing significantly from the more commonly known pancreatic adenocarcinoma. PNETs arise from the islet cells of the pancreas, which are responsible for producing hormones that regulate blood sugar levels. These tumors can be either functional, secreting hormones that lead to clinical syndromes, or non-functional, which do not produce hormones and often remain undiagnosed until they grow large enough to cause symptoms by mass effect.

Functional PNETs can lead to a variety of symptoms depending on the type of hormone they secrete, including insulinomas (excess insulin), gastrinomas (excess gastrin), and glucagonomas (excess glucagon), each associated with distinct clinical syndromes such as hypoglycemia, Zollinger-Ellison syndrome, and necrolytic migratory erythema, respectively.

The rarity of PNETs poses challenges in diagnosis and treatment. Imaging studies, biochemical tests, and biopsy are key to diagnosis, with treatment options including surgery, targeted therapy, hormone therapy, chemotherapy, and peptide receptor radionuclide therapy (PRRT) for certain types.

Despite their challenges, advancements in understanding and treating PNETs have improved outcomes and quality of life for patients. Personalized treatment strategies, based on the tumor's characteristics and the patient's condition, are essential for managing these complex tumors.

Genetic and Congenital Pancreatic Conditions

Genetic and congenital pancreatic conditions represent a complex group of disorders that can significantly impact pancreatic function and overall health from an early age. These conditions often stem from genetic mutations passed down through families or developmental anomalies occurring during fetal development. Examples include hereditary pancreatitis, cystic fibrosis, and congenital pancreatic anomalies like pancreatic divisum.

Hereditary pancreatitis is characterized by recurrent episodes of pancreatitis, typically beginning in childhood, due to mutations in specific genes such as PRSS1. This condition significantly increases the risk of developing chronic pancreatitis and pancreatic cancer later in life. Management focuses on symptom control, lifestyle modifications, and monitoring for complications.

Cystic fibrosis, caused by mutations in the CFTR gene, leads to the production of thick mucus that can block pancreatic ducts, inhibiting the secretion of digestive enzymes and leading to malabsorption and nutritional deficiencies. Treatment includes enzyme replacement therapy and nutritional support.

Pancreatic divisum, the most common congenital pancreatic anomaly, occurs when the ductal systems of the pancreas fail to fuse properly during fetal development. This condition may be asymptomatic or lead to recurrent pancreatitis in some individuals.

Management of these genetic and congenital conditions requires a multidisciplinary approach, including genetic counseling, specialized medical care, and supportive therapies to address symptoms and prevent complications.

Innovative Therapies and Hope on the Horizon

The landscape of treatment for pancreatic diseases is rapidly evolving, offering new hope and innovative therapies to patients facing these challenging conditions. Breakthroughs in research and technology are paving the way for more effective and targeted treatments, significantly improving outcomes and quality of life.

One promising area is the development of targeted therapies for pancreatic cancer, which aim to attack specific genetic mutations or pathways involved in tumor growth. For example, drugs targeting the KRAS mutation, present in a significant portion of pancreatic cancers, are showing promise in clinical trials. Additionally, immunotherapy, which harnesses the body's immune system to fight cancer, is emerging as a potential treatment for certain patients with pancreatic cancer, especially those with specific biomarkers.

For chronic pancreatitis and pancreatic insufficiency, enzyme replacement therapies are becoming more sophisticated, with new formulations designed for better absorption and patient compliance. Islet cell transplantation is another area of interest, offering potential for patients with chronic pancreatitis to regain insulin production and reduce the risk of diabetes.

Moreover, advances in endoscopic and minimally invasive surgical techniques are improving the management of pancreatic cysts and pseudocysts, reducing recovery times and enhancing patient outcomes.

These innovative therapies, alongside ongoing research into the genetic and molecular underpinnings of pancreatic diseases, signal a future where personalized medicine could significantly impact treatment strategies, offering hope and improved prospects for those affected.

Chapter 9

The Emotional Journey

The Psychological Impact of Chronic Illness

The emotional journey of living with a chronic illness like pancreatic disease encompasses a wide range of psychological challenges that can profoundly affect an individual's mental health and well-being. The initial diagnosis often brings a wave of shock, fear, and uncertainty, as patients and their families grapple with the implications of a long-term condition that may significantly alter life's trajectory.

As the reality of the diagnosis settles in, individuals may experience a rollercoaster of emotions, including sadness, anger, and frustration, stemming from the physical limitations, pain, and the need for ongoing treatment. The chronic nature of pancreatic diseases, with their unpredictable flare-ups and impact on daily activities, can lead to feelings of loss of control and independence, contributing to anxiety and depression.

Moreover, the social and financial implications of chronic illness can exacerbate stress, as individuals may face difficulties in maintaining employment, managing medical expenses, and fulfilling social roles. Isolation and withdrawal from social activities are common, as the effort to manage symptoms and treatment regimens can overshadow other aspects of life.

Recognizing and addressing these emotional and psychological challenges are crucial components of comprehensive care. Support from mental health professionals, support groups, and a strong network of friends and family can provide essential emotional scaffolding, helping individuals navigate the complex emotional landscape of chronic illness.

Strategies for Mental Health: From Therapy to Mindfulness

Strategies for maintaining and enhancing mental health in the face of chronic illness are diverse, spanning from professional therapy to self-directed practices like mindfulness. Therapy, particularly cognitive-behavioral therapy (CBT), offers a structured approach to addressing the psychological impacts of chronic diseases, such as anxiety and depression. It helps individuals develop coping strategies, challenge negative thought patterns, and build resilience against the emotional toll of their condition.

Mindfulness and meditation have also emerged as powerful tools for mental health management. These practices encourage individuals to focus on the present moment, cultivating an attitude of acceptance and reducing stress. By practicing mindfulness, patients can gain a greater sense of control over their emotional responses to pain and illness, mitigating feelings of helplessness and despair.

Support groups, whether in-person or online, provide a sense of community and understanding that can be incredibly therapeutic. Sharing experiences and strategies with others facing similar challenges can lessen feelings of isolation and provide practical advice for managing the condition.

Incorporating regular physical activity, when possible, serves as another effective strategy for improving mental health. Exercise can reduce symptoms of depression and anxiety, enhance mood, and improve overall physical well-being, creating a positive feedback loop that supports both physical and mental health in the context of chronic illness.

Building Your Support Network

Building a robust support network is crucial for individuals navigating the complexities of chronic illnesses, including pancreatic diseases. This network can comprise family members, friends, healthcare professionals, and peers facing similar health challenges. A well-rounded support system provides emotional comfort, practical assistance, and valuable information, contributing significantly to managing the disease's physical and psychological aspects.

Family and friends play a pivotal role, offering day-to-day support, understanding, and companionship. They can help with practical tasks, such as attending medical appointments or managing household chores, alleviating some of the burdens associated with the illness.

Healthcare professionals, including doctors, nurses, and therapists, form another essential layer of support. They offer expert advice, treatment options, and emotional counseling to help patients navigate their health journey. Establishing open communication with this team ensures that care is tailored to the individual's needs and preferences.

Peer support groups, whether found through local communities or online platforms, provide a unique space for sharing experiences and coping strategies. These groups offer empathy, encouragement, and insights from others who truly understand the challenges of living with a chronic illness.

Actively cultivating these relationships and resources can empower individuals to manage their health more effectively, fostering resilience and a sense of community that enriches their journey towards well-being.

Chapter 10

Living with Pancreatic Disease

Dietary Guidelines and Nutritional Support

Living with pancreatic diseases, such as chronic pancreatitis, pancreatic insufficiency, or pancreatic cancer, necessitates careful attention to dietary guidelines and nutritional support. The pancreas plays a vital role in digestion by producing enzymes that break down food. When the pancreas is compromised, as in these conditions, proper nutrition becomes a central focus to maintain overall health.

1. Low-Fat Diet: A common recommendation for individuals with pancreatic diseases is to follow a low-fat diet. This helps reduce the workload on the pancreas, as

it struggles to produce digestive enzymes. Limiting dietary fat can alleviate symptoms like abdominal pain, diarrhea, and steatorrhea (fatty stools).

2. Small, Frequent Meals: Eating smaller, more frequent meals throughout the day can ease the digestive process and minimize discomfort. This approach prevents overloading the pancreas and provides a steadier release of enzymes.

3. Enzyme Replacement Therapy (ERT): For those with pancreatic insufficiency, enzyme supplements are prescribed to assist in the digestion of fats, proteins, and carbohydrates. These enzymes should be taken with every meal and snack to ensure proper nutrient absorption.

4. Balanced Nutrition: Maintaining a balanced diet is essential to prevent nutritional deficiencies. A diet rich in lean proteins, complex carbohydrates, and a variety of fruits and vegetables is recommended. Special attention should be given to consuming enough protein and calories to prevent weight loss and muscle wasting.

5. Hydration: Staying well-hydrated is crucial, especially for individuals experiencing diarrhea. Dehydration can worsen symptoms and lead to additional complications.

6. Vitamin and Mineral Supplements: In some cases, supplements may be necessary to address specific nutrient deficiencies. Fat-soluble vitamins (A, D, E, and K) may need to be supplemented, as these are often poorly absorbed without proper pancreatic function.

7. Consultation with a Dietitian: Working with a registered dietitian who specializes in pancreatic diseases can be invaluable. They can create a personalized meal plan tailored to the individual's specific needs and provide ongoing guidance and support.

8. Patient Education: Understanding one's condition and how diet affects it is crucial. Patients should be educated about their dietary restrictions, medication management, and symptom monitoring to empower them in their daily lives.

By following these dietary guidelines and seeking nutritional support, individuals living with pancreatic diseases can enhance their quality of life, alleviate symptoms, and better manage their condition. It's a vital component of comprehensive care that contributes to overall well-being.

Exercise and Physical Well-being

Incorporating exercise into the daily routine is beneficial for individuals living with pancreatic diseases, as it can significantly contribute to physical well-being and overall health. While the ability to engage in exercise may vary based on the specific condition and its severity, there are adaptable strategies to consider:

1. Consultation with Healthcare Providers: Before starting any exercise regimen, it's essential to consult with healthcare providers, including gastroenterologists and physical therapists, who can provide guidance tailored to the individual's condition. They can help determine the appropriate level of exercise and any precautions needed.

2. Low-Impact Activities: For many with pancreatic diseases, especially those with chronic pain or compromised physical health, low-impact activities such as walking, swimming, or stationary cycling can be gentle yet effective ways to stay active. These exercises minimize strain on the body while promoting cardiovascular health and muscle strength.

3. Yoga and Stretching: Yoga and stretching routines can improve flexibility, reduce muscle tension, and enhance

overall physical comfort. Modified yoga poses and gentle stretching exercises can be adapted to accommodate different physical abilities.

4. Breathing Exercises: Practicing deep breathing exercises can help manage pain and stress. Techniques like diaphragmatic breathing promote relaxation and can be integrated into daily routines.

5. Regular Physical Activity: Consistency is key. Establishing a routine that includes regular physical activity, even in shorter intervals, can contribute to improved endurance and overall well-being.

6. Emphasis on Balance and Posture: Specific exercises targeting balance and posture can be particularly helpful for those with pancreatic diseases. Improved balance can reduce the risk of falls and injuries.

7. Pain Management: For individuals dealing with chronic pain, it's crucial to manage pain effectively with the help of healthcare providers. Adequate pain management can make exercise more feasible and enjoyable.

Regular physical activity not only supports physical well-being but also contributes to emotional and mental health. Exercise releases endorphins, which can improve mood and reduce stress, helping individuals better cope with the challenges of living with a chronic illness. It's essential to approach exercise with a personalized plan that takes into account individual health status, preferences, and any limitations imposed by the specific pancreatic disease.

Integrating Medical Care into Daily Life

Integrating medical care into daily life is essential for individuals living with pancreatic diseases. These conditions often require ongoing monitoring, medication management, and regular medical appointments. Here are some strategies to seamlessly incorporate medical care into daily routines:

1. Medication Management: Adhering to medication schedules is crucial. Set daily alarms or reminders to take prescribed medications, especially for enzyme replacements or pain management. Keep a medication diary to track dosages and any side effects.

2. Meal Planning: Meal planning can simplify dietary requirements. Prepare and store enzyme supplements, snacks, and low-fat meals in advance to ensure they are readily available throughout the day.

3. Hydration: Stay hydrated, which is vital for overall health. Keep a water bottle within reach, and aim to drink fluids consistently to prevent dehydration, a common issue in some pancreatic diseases.

4. Symptom Journal: Maintain a symptom journal to track changes in health, including pain levels, digestive symptoms, and emotional well-being. This journal can serve as a valuable resource during medical appointments, aiding healthcare providers in adjusting treatment plans.

5. Supportive Devices: If required, use supportive devices such as orthopedic cushions or mobility aids to enhance comfort and mobility, making daily activities more manageable.

6. Communication: Maintain open communication with healthcare providers. Discuss any changes in symptoms, side effects of medications, or concerns promptly. Regularly scheduled check-ups ensure that the disease is well-managed.

7. Self-Care Routine: Prioritize self-care, including stress reduction techniques, relaxation exercises, and mindfulness practices. Incorporate these into daily routines to foster emotional well-being.

8. Physical Activity: If possible, include gentle physical activity into daily life, as recommended by healthcare providers. Even short walks or stretching exercises can make a significant difference in overall health.

9. Support Network: Engage family and friends in the process. Share information about the condition, treatment plans, and dietary restrictions, enabling them to provide valuable support and understanding.

Integrating medical care into daily life requires organization, commitment, and a proactive approach. By creating a structured routine that incorporates medical needs and supports overall well-being, individuals with pancreatic diseases can effectively manage their condition while maintaining a fulfilling and balanced life.

Chapter 11

Beyond the Patient

Advice for Caregivers: How to Support Your Loved One

Supporting a loved one with a pancreatic disease can be emotionally and physically demanding. Caregivers play a crucial role in their loved one's journey to manage the condition effectively and maintain their overall well-being. Here are some pieces of advice for caregivers:

1. Educate Yourself: Learn about the specific pancreatic disease your loved one is facing. Understanding the condition, its symptoms, treatment options, and dietary restrictions will enable you to provide informed support.

2. Open Communication: Foster open and empathetic communication. Encourage your loved one to share their feelings, concerns, and needs. Be a good listener and provide emotional support.

3. Accompany to Appointments: Attend medical appointments with your loved one when possible. Take notes, ask questions, and ensure that both you and your loved one fully understand the treatment plan and any recommended lifestyle changes.

4. Assist with Medication: Help your loved one manage their medication schedule. Set reminders, organize pillboxes, and ensure that medications are taken as prescribed.

5. Meal Preparation: Assist with meal planning and preparation, especially if dietary restrictions are involved. Focus on creating low-fat, nutritious meals that align with their dietary needs.

6. Provide Emotional Support: Be there as a source of emotional support. Offer encouragement, empathy, and a listening ear during difficult moments. Help them navigate the emotional challenges of living with a chronic illness.

7. Encourage Physical Activity: Encourage gentle physical activity as recommended by healthcare providers. Offer to accompany your loved one on walks or to physical therapy sessions.

8. Respite Care: Remember to take care of yourself too. Caregiving can be demanding, so don't hesitate to seek respite care or support from others when needed to prevent burnout.

9. Support Network: Encourage your loved one to connect with support groups or therapy services for emotional and psychological support. Offer to help them find these resources if necessary.

10. Celebrate Achievements: Acknowledge and celebrate your loved one's achievements, no matter how small they may seem. Living with a pancreatic disease can be challenging, and positive reinforcement can boost morale.

Above all, caregiving is a partnership. Approach it with patience, empathy, and a commitment to helping your loved one manage their condition effectively while maintaining their quality of life. Your support can make a significant difference in their journey.

Navigating the Healthcare System: Insurance, Costs, and Assistance

Navigating the healthcare system, including insurance, costs, and available assistance programs, is essential for individuals living with pancreatic diseases. Managing the financial aspects of healthcare can be complex, but it's crucial for ensuring access to necessary treatments and services:

1. Health Insurance: Understand the specifics of your health insurance policy, including coverage for doctor visits, medications, procedures, and hospital stays. Be aware of any pre-authorization requirements and in-network providers to minimize out-of-pocket expenses.

2. Costs and Co-Payments: Be prepared for out-of-pocket costs, such as co-payments, deductibles, and co-insurance. Budget for these expenses and keep track of medical bills to ensure accuracy.

3. Prior Authorization: In some cases, certain treatments or medications may require prior authorization from the insurance company. Work closely with healthcare providers to facilitate this process.

4. Prescription Coverage: Familiarize yourself with your prescription drug coverage. Ensure that necessary medications, including enzyme replacements or pain management drugs, are covered, and explore generic options if available.

5. Assistance Programs: Investigate government assistance programs, nonprofit organizations, and pharmaceutical assistance programs that may help cover the costs of medications and treatments. Some programs provide financial support based on income and need.

6. Medical Billing Advocacy: Consider enlisting the help of a medical billing advocate or a patient advocacy organization if you encounter billing issues, denied claims, or excessive charges. They can assist in resolving disputes and reducing healthcare costs.

7. Financial Planning: Work with a financial advisor or counselor to create a healthcare financial plan. This can include budgeting for medical expenses and exploring options for long-term financial security.

8. Appeals Process: If insurance claims are denied, understand the appeals process and your rights as a patient. Be prepared to provide necessary documentation and information to support your case.

9. Patient Assistance Hotlines: Many healthcare organizations and insurance companies offer patient assistance hotlines to address billing and insurance inquiries. These resources can be valuable for resolving issues promptly.

10. Documentation: Keep detailed records of medical expenses, insurance correspondence, and medical receipts. These records can be crucial for tax deductions and verifying billing accuracy.

Navigating the healthcare system can be challenging, but with careful planning, advocacy, and utilization of available resources, individuals with pancreatic diseases can effectively manage their healthcare expenses and access the necessary treatments and support.

Legal and Ethical Considerations in Care

Legal and ethical considerations play a vital role in providing care for individuals living with pancreatic diseases. Healthcare providers, caregivers, and patients themselves should be aware of these considerations to ensure the best possible care and protection of patients' rights.

1. Informed Consent: Healthcare providers must obtain informed consent from patients before any medical procedure or treatment. Patients should be fully informed about the risks, benefits, and alternatives, allowing them to make informed decisions about their care.

2. Patient Privacy: Protecting patient privacy and confidentiality is essential. Health information should be kept secure and only shared with authorized individuals. Healthcare providers must adhere to laws like the Health Insurance Portability and Accountability Act (HIPAA) in the United States.

3. Advance Directives: Patients have the right to create advance directives, such as living wills and healthcare proxies, to outline their preferences for medical treatment in case they become unable to make decisions. Healthcare providers should respect these directives.

4. End-of-Life Care: Ethical considerations surrounding end-of-life care, such as palliative care and hospice, should be addressed respectfully and in accordance with the patient's wishes.

5. Pain Management: Ethical considerations related to pain management include ensuring that patients receive adequate pain relief while avoiding overmedication and

opioid addiction. Balancing pain control and potential side effects is essential.

6. Cultural Competence: Healthcare providers must be culturally competent, respecting patients' cultural and religious beliefs and tailoring care accordingly.

7. Quality of Life: Ethical decisions often involve weighing the potential benefits and burdens of medical treatments on the patient's overall quality of life. Shared decision-making between patients, caregivers, and healthcare providers is crucial.

8. Access to Care: Legal and ethical considerations also extend to ensuring equitable access to care. All patients should have access to appropriate treatments and support, regardless of their socioeconomic status or other factors.

9. Advance Research: Ethical guidelines must be followed in medical research involving patients with pancreatic diseases, including obtaining informed consent and protecting participants' rights.

10. Euthanasia and Assisted Suicide: In some regions, legal and ethical debates surround euthanasia and assisted suicide. These complex issues require careful consideration of the patient's autonomy and quality of life.

Navigating these legal and ethical considerations requires collaboration and communication among healthcare providers, patients, caregivers, and legal professionals to ensure that care is both medically sound and ethically justifiable, respecting patients' rights and autonomy throughout their healthcare journey.

Chapter 12

The Power of Community

Finding and Engaging with Support Groups

The power of community, especially through support groups, is invaluable for individuals living with pancreatic diseases. These groups provide a sense of belonging, understanding, and emotional support that can profoundly impact the journey of both patients and caregivers. Here's how to find and engage with support groups effectively:

1. Online Resources: Start by exploring online platforms, such as social media, forums, and websites dedicated to pancreatic diseases. These virtual communities offer a

convenient way to connect with others who share similar experiences.

2. Medical Facilities: Many hospitals and healthcare institutions host support groups specifically for patients with pancreatic diseases. Inquire with your healthcare provider or local hospital to find information about local groups.

3. Nonprofit Organizations: Pancreatic disease-focused nonprofit organizations often facilitate support groups and provide resources. These organizations can guide you to local meetings or virtual gatherings.

4. Patient Advocacy Groups: Organizations like the Pancreatic Cancer Action Network (PanCAN) and the National Pancreas Foundation offer a wealth of resources, including support groups, educational materials, and events.

5. Social Media: Social networking platforms like Facebook and Reddit host numerous groups and communities where individuals can share their experiences and find support.

6. Local Community Centers: Check with local community centers or libraries for information about support groups in your area. Some groups may host in-

person meetings, while others may offer virtual gatherings.

Engaging with support groups can provide numerous benefits. Participants can exchange practical advice on managing symptoms, dietary tips, and coping strategies. Moreover, these communities offer a safe space to express emotions, share stories, and find inspiration from others' journeys.

Active participation in support groups fosters a sense of empowerment, reduces isolation, and helps individuals gain a better understanding of their condition. By connecting with others who face similar challenges, patients and caregivers can navigate the complexities of pancreatic diseases with renewed hope and resilience.

Online Resources and Social Networks

Online resources and social networks play a crucial role in the lives of individuals living with pancreatic diseases and their caregivers. In today's digital age, these platforms provide a wealth of information, support, and connectivity, helping to navigate the complexities of these conditions:

1. Information and Education: The internet offers a vast repository of educational materials, articles, and research about pancreatic diseases. Patients and caregivers can access up-to-date information to better understand their condition, treatment options, and management strategies.

2. Support Communities: Online forums, social media groups, and dedicated websites provide a sense of community for those affected by pancreatic diseases. These virtual spaces allow individuals to connect with others facing similar challenges, share experiences, and offer emotional support.

3. Telehealth and Telemedicine: Online platforms enable remote consultations with healthcare providers, making it easier for patients to access medical advice and treatment without the need for frequent in-person visits.

4. Advocacy and Awareness: Nonprofit organizations, patient advocacy groups, and social media campaigns use online platforms to raise awareness about pancreatic diseases, advocate for research funding, and provide resources for patients and caregivers.

5. Lifestyle and Dietary Guidance: Websites and apps offer tools for managing dietary restrictions, tracking symptoms, and adhering to treatment plans. These

resources empower individuals to make informed lifestyle choices.

6. Emotional Support: Online mental health resources, including therapy platforms and support groups, can help individuals cope with the emotional challenges of living with a chronic illness.

7. Global Connectivity: Online platforms facilitate connections with individuals from around the world, allowing patients and caregivers to access a diverse range of experiences, treatment approaches, and cultural perspectives.

It's essential to approach online resources with discernment, verifying information from reliable sources and consulting with healthcare providers when necessary. By harnessing the power of online resources and social networks, individuals affected by pancreatic diseases can access a wealth of knowledge, support, and opportunities for improved well-being and quality of life.

Chapter 13

Looking Forward

Advances in Pancreatic Disease Research

Looking forward, there is reason for hope and optimism in the field of pancreatic disease research. Advances in medical science and technology continue to drive progress in understanding and managing these conditions.

1. Early Detection: Researchers are working on improving early detection methods for pancreatic diseases, including the development of blood tests and imaging techniques that can identify issues at earlier, more treatable stages.

2. Targeted Therapies: Targeted therapies for pancreatic cancer are a promising avenue. Scientists are exploring drugs that specifically target genetic mutations and pathways involved in tumor growth, potentially leading to more effective treatments.

3. Immunotherapy: Immunotherapy is emerging as a potential treatment for pancreatic cancer. This approach harnesses the body's immune system to attack cancer cells, offering new hope for patients.

4. Personalized Medicine: The era of personalized medicine is taking hold. Genetic profiling of pancreatic tumors allows for tailored treatment plans, optimizing outcomes for individual patients.

5. Enzyme Replacement: Research continues to refine enzyme replacement therapies for pancreatic insufficiency, with a focus on improving enzyme formulations and delivery methods.

6. Minimally Invasive Procedures: Advances in minimally invasive surgical techniques are reducing the invasiveness and recovery times for procedures related to pancreatic diseases.

7. Patient-Centered Care: A growing emphasis on patient-centered care means that treatment plans are

increasingly tailored to the unique needs and preferences of each patient.

8. Regenerative Medicine: Regenerative medicine approaches, including stem cell therapy, hold potential for repairing damaged pancreatic tissue in chronic pancreatitis.

9. Patient Empowerment: Patients are becoming more informed and engaged in their healthcare, contributing to improved outcomes and research efforts.

While challenges remain, the collaborative efforts of researchers, healthcare professionals, and advocacy groups offer promise for a brighter future in the fight against pancreatic diseases. These advances are not only extending lives but also improving the quality of life for those affected by these conditions.

Advocacy and Raising Awareness

Advocacy and raising awareness are essential components of the fight against pancreatic diseases. These efforts play a pivotal role in driving research, improving patient care, and ultimately saving lives.

1. Research Funding: Advocacy groups and individuals raise their voices to urge governments and institutions to allocate more funding for pancreatic disease research. Increased research funding is vital for discovering new treatments, early detection methods, and potential cures.

2. Support for Patients: Advocacy efforts often result in improved support services for patients and their families. This includes access to information, support groups, and financial assistance programs.

3. Early Detection Campaigns: Raising awareness about the importance of early detection through educational campaigns can lead to more individuals seeking medical attention at the first signs of pancreatic diseases, potentially improving outcomes.

4. Pushing for Policy Change: Advocacy groups work tirelessly to influence policy changes that benefit patients. This includes advocating for healthcare reform, insurance coverage, and patient rights.

5. Stigma Reduction: Raising awareness helps reduce the stigma associated with pancreatic diseases. This encourages open dialogue, support, and understanding within communities.

6. Supporting Research Initiatives: Advocacy groups often support specific research initiatives, clinical trials, and collaborations that aim to find innovative solutions for pancreatic diseases.

7. Community Engagement: Through events, walks, and fundraisers, advocacy groups and individuals engage with their communities to educate and raise funds for research and patient support.

8. Global Impact: Pancreatic disease awareness is not limited to one region; it's a global effort. International collaborations and awareness campaigns contribute to the global fight against these diseases.

Advocacy and awareness efforts are fueled by the determination of patients, caregivers, healthcare professionals, and organizations committed to making a difference. By amplifying their voices and sharing their stories, these advocates are working towards a future where pancreatic diseases are better understood, more effectively treated, and ultimately prevented.

Contributing to the Fight: How You Can Help

Contributing to the fight against pancreatic diseases is a meaningful endeavor that can make a significant impact on the lives of patients and the advancement of research and support. Here are ways in which you can help:

1. Donate to Research: Consider donating to reputable research organizations and foundations dedicated to pancreatic disease research. Your contributions can support groundbreaking studies and innovative treatments.

2. Participate in Clinical Trials: If you are eligible, participating in clinical trials can help researchers test new therapies and treatments. Clinical trial participants play a crucial role in advancing medical knowledge.

3. Raise Awareness: Use your voice and social media platforms to raise awareness about pancreatic diseases. Share informative articles, personal stories, and advocacy initiatives to educate others.

4. Fundraise: Organize fundraising events, such as charity walks, runs, or online campaigns, to support

research and patient care. Encourage friends and family to join or donate.

5. Volunteer: Offer your time and expertise to local or national organizations dedicated to pancreatic diseases. Volunteer opportunities can include event planning, patient support, or advocacy work.

6. Support Patients: Provide emotional support and assistance to individuals and families affected by pancreatic diseases. Offering a helping hand or a listening ear can make a meaningful difference.

7. Advocate for Policy Change: Get involved in advocacy efforts to influence policies related to pancreatic diseases. Write to your elected representatives and attend advocacy events to promote positive change.

8. Educate Yourself: Stay informed about the latest developments in pancreatic disease research and treatment. Knowledge is a powerful tool for advocacy and support.

9. Join Support Groups: If you or a loved one is affected by pancreatic diseases, consider joining support groups to connect with others facing similar challenges. Sharing experiences can provide comfort and insights.

10. Remember Loved Ones: Honor the memory of those who have lost their lives to pancreatic diseases by supporting initiatives that aim to prevent and treat these conditions.

Every contribution, no matter how small, can help further the fight against pancreatic diseases. By working together, we can improve patient outcomes, raise awareness, and make a lasting impact on the lives of those affected by these conditions.

Appendices

Appendix A: Nutritional Resources and Recipe Ideas

Proper nutrition plays a pivotal role in managing pancreatic diseases. This appendix provides a comprehensive list of nutritional resources and a selection of recipe ideas tailored to the dietary needs and restrictions associated with pancreatic diseases.

Nutritional Resources:

1. Registered Dietitian: Consult with a registered dietitian who specializes in pancreatic diseases. They can create personalized meal plans and provide dietary guidance tailored to your specific condition.

2. National Pancreas Foundation (NPF): The NPF offers educational materials, including dietary guidelines and nutritional advice, to support individuals with pancreatic

diseases. Visit their website or contact them for resources.

3. Cookbooks: Explore cookbooks designed for individuals with pancreatic diseases or those requiring low-fat, easily digestible recipes. Look for titles like "Pancreatitis Diet Cookbook" or "Low-Fat Pancreatic Recipes."

4. Online Resources: Numerous websites and blogs offer nutritional advice, meal planning tips, and recipes suitable for pancreatic disease management. Be sure to verify the credibility of the sources.

5. Support Groups: Join online or in-person support groups for individuals with pancreatic diseases. Members often share dietary tips and recipes that have worked well for them.

Recipe Ideas:

1. Easy-to-Digest Smoothies: Blend low-fat yogurt, banana, honey, and a handful of berries for a nutritious and easy-to-digest breakfast or snack.

2. Mashed Potatoes: Prepare mashed potatoes with low-fat milk and a touch of butter for a creamy and comforting side dish.

3. Baked Chicken: Season skinless, boneless chicken breast with herbs and bake it with a drizzle of olive oil for a protein-rich and low-fat main course.

4. Vegetable Soup: Create a vegetable soup with carrots, zucchini, and spinach, using a low-sodium vegetable broth for flavor.

5. Quinoa Salad: Make a quinoa salad with diced cucumbers, tomatoes, and parsley, dressed with lemon juice and a touch of olive oil.

6. Oatmeal with Apples: Cook oatmeal with diced apples and a sprinkle of cinnamon for a fiber-rich and satisfying breakfast.

7. Baked Salmon: Season salmon fillets with lemon and herbs, then bake them for a heart-healthy source of omega-3 fatty acids.

8. Fruit Salad: Prepare a fruit salad with ripe melon, berries, and grapes for a refreshing and vitamin-packed dessert.

9. Steamed Vegetables: Steam broccoli, cauliflower, and carrots for a nutrient-rich side dish that is easy on the digestive system.

10. Low-Fat Pudding: Enjoy a small portion of low-fat pudding for a sweet treat that doesn't compromise dietary restrictions.

Remember to consult with your healthcare provider or registered dietitian before making significant dietary changes. These resources and recipe ideas are meant to support your nutritional needs and enhance your overall well-being while living with pancreatic diseases.

Appendix B: Glossary of Terms

Certainly, here's a glossary of terms for your book on pancreatic diseases:

A

1. Abdominal Pain: Discomfort or tenderness in the area between the chest and the pelvis, often associated with pancreatic diseases.

B

2. Bilirubin: A yellow pigment produced during the breakdown of red blood cells, which can accumulate and cause jaundice when the pancreatic duct is blocked.

C

3. Chronic Pancreatitis: Ongoing inflammation of the pancreas that can lead to permanent damage and digestive problems.

D

4. Diabetes Mellitus: A condition characterized by high blood sugar levels, which can result from pancreatic diseases affecting insulin production.

5. Digestive Enzymes: Proteins produced by the pancreas that help break down food in the digestive system.

6. Endoscopic Retrograde Cholangiopancreatography (ERCP): A procedure used to diagnose and treat disorders of the bile ducts and pancreas.

E

7. Enzyme Replacement Therapy (ERT): Treatment for pancreatic insufficiency involving the use of pancreatic enzyme supplements to aid digestion.

G

8. Gastrointestinal Bleeding: The presence of blood in the digestive tract, which can occur in some pancreatic diseases.

I

9. Immunotherapy: A cancer treatment that uses the body's immune system to target and destroy cancer cells.

10. Jaundice: Yellowing of the skin and eyes due to the buildup of bilirubin, often a sign of pancreatic disease.

N

11. Nutritional Deficiencies: Insufficient intake or absorption of essential nutrients, common in pancreatic diseases.

P

12. Pancreatic Cancer: A type of cancer that begins in the pancreas and can spread to other parts of the body.

13. Pancreatectomy: Surgical removal of all or part of the pancreas.

14. Pancreatic Duct: A tube that carries digestive enzymes and other substances from the pancreas to the small intestine.

15. Pancreatic Insufficiency: Inadequate production of digestive enzymes by the pancreas.

16. Pancreatic Pseudocyst: A collection of fluid that can form in or around the pancreas after inflammation or injury.

S

17. Steatorrhea: The passage of pale, bulky, and foul-smelling stools, often a symptom of pancreatic insufficiency.

T

18. Total Parenteral Nutrition (TPN): A method of feeding that provides all nutrients intravenously, used in severe cases of malnutrition.

This glossary provides definitions for key terms related to pancreatic diseases, helping readers better understand the content of your book and the medical terminology associated with these conditions.

Appendix C: Directory of Support Services

and Resources

Directory of Support Services and Resources

In this directory, you will find a comprehensive list of support services and valuable resources tailored to individuals and families affected by pancreatic diseases. These resources are designed to provide assistance, information, and emotional support throughout your journey with pancreatic diseases. Please note that this directory is not exhaustive, and it's advisable to verify the availability and suitability of these resources for your specific needs.

1. National Pancreas Foundation (NPF)

- Website: [www.pancreasfoundation.org](https://pancreasfoundation.org/)
- Contact: [Contact NPF](https://pancreasfoundation.org/contact/)

The NPF is a nonprofit organization dedicated to supporting individuals with pancreatic diseases. They offer educational materials, research updates, and information about local support groups.

2. Patient Support Groups

- Various online and in-person support groups provide a sense of community and a platform for sharing experiences with others facing similar challenges. Search for local groups or explore online communities dedicated to pancreatic diseases.

3. Registered Dietitians

- Consult a registered dietitian with expertise in pancreatic diseases for personalized dietary guidance and meal planning. They can help you navigate dietary restrictions and optimize your nutrition.

4. Local Healthcare Providers

- Your local healthcare facilities, including hospitals, clinics, and specialty centers, can provide access to medical professionals experienced in the treatment of pancreatic diseases.

5. Clinical Trials

- Clinical trials offer opportunities to participate in cutting-edge research and potentially access innovative treatments. Speak with your healthcare provider about available trials.

6. Financial Assistance Programs

- Some organizations and foundations provide financial assistance to individuals and families facing the financial burden of medical expenses related to pancreatic diseases. Explore options that may be available to you.

7. Palliative Care Services

- Palliative care teams focus on improving your quality of life and managing symptoms, especially in advanced cases. Inquire about palliative care services at your healthcare facility.

8. Mental Health Services

- Seeking the support of mental health professionals or therapists can help you cope with the emotional challenges associated with chronic illness. Consider therapy or counseling services.

9. Pancreatic Disease Research Organizations

- Connect with organizations dedicated to funding research on pancreatic diseases. They often provide updates on the latest research and opportunities for involvement.

10. Insurance and Financial Advisors

- Insurance and financial advisors can assist you in navigating the complexities of healthcare coverage, medical bills, and financial planning during your journey with pancreatic diseases.

Note: The availability of these resources may vary by location and individual circumstances. It is advisable to consult with your healthcare provider or a trusted medical professional for guidance on accessing and utilizing these services effectively.

This directory is intended to serve as a starting point in your quest for information and support. Please reach out to the listed resources and professionals to explore the services that align with your specific needs and goals.